essential careers ™

A CAREER AS A
PHYSICAL
THERAPIST

THERESE HARASYMIW

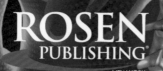

ROSEN
PUBLISHING

NEW YORK

For Mark, the best therapist I know

Published in 2011 by The Rosen Publishing Group, Inc.
29 East 21st Street, New York, NY 10010

Copyright © 2011 by The Rosen Publishing Group, Inc.

First Edition

Library of Congress Cataloging-in-Publication Data

Harasymiw, Therese.
A career as a physical therapist / Therese Harasymiw.—1st ed.
    p. cm.—(Essential careers)
Includes bibliographical references and index.
ISBN 978-1-4358-9467-9 (library binding)
1. Physical therapists—Vocational guidance—Popular works. I. Title.
RM705.H37 2011
615.8'2023—dc22

2009045009

Manufactured in the United States of America

CPSIA Compliance Information: Batch #S10YA: For further information, contact Rosen Publishing, New York, New York, at 1-800-237-9932.

contents

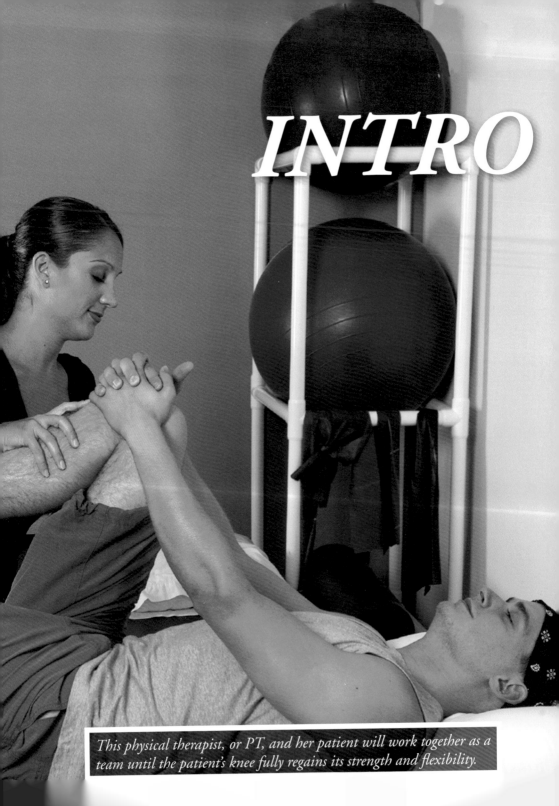

INTRO

This physical therapist, or PT, and her patient will work together as a team until the patient's knee fully regains its strength and flexibility.

DUCTION

The career of a physical therapist requires knowing the inner workings of the human body. It involves helping people as young as newborns and as old as great-grandparents. It might mean working with a famous football player one day and a neighbor the next day. All of these things are possible with a career in physical therapy.

Physical therapists, called physiotherapists in Canada and some other countries, are health care professionals who evaluate and treat health problems. Specifically, they help improve people's ability to move and function in their daily lives. A familiar role of a physical therapist, or PT, is to aid someone who has broken a bone. A doctor repositions the bone and makes sure it cannot move until it heals properly. However, after it has healed, the injured limb may have lost its strength and flexibility. A physical therapist can help a patient regain the limb's former abilities.

Physical therapists can teach others how to make their bones, muscles, joints, and other body parts strong and flexible. They can recommend treatments that will soothe aches and pains after a patient has undergone surgery. They can tell someone when to push his or her body and when to let it rest. They may use tools, machines, or their own bodies to accomplish their tasks. They can help someone learn to live more comfortably with a disease or disorder. These are just some parts of a physical therapist's job.

Physical therapy is a career in demand. PTs are a vital and growing part of the health care workforce. This demand

and growth makes physical therapy an essential career. This means that it's recession-proof, or not significantly affected by a recession or a period in which fewer people have financial prosperity. A recession is shorter and less severe than a depression. In both, people have difficulty finding jobs and, as a result, have difficulty paying their bills. They don't have as much money to spend on themselves or on others.

Certain careers suffer during a recession. Jobs that rely on people having money to spend, such as those in the travel and entertainment industries, are not a dependable source of income during an economic downturn. Often, people are not hired for these jobs, and sometimes they are even laid off from such jobs during a recession. Other careers are recession-proof because people will always need certain services. Education and law enforcement are examples of recession-proof careers. Communities will always need teachers and police officers.

Massage is just one of many treatments a physical therapist may use in helping a patient reduce pain and stiffness. Years of education help PTs discern the best treatment for each patient.

Similarly, health care is a necessity, so health care careers, including physical therapy, are considered recession-proof as well.

Job stability during tough economic times is one thing to consider when choosing a career. Perhaps just as important is job satisfaction. In many surveys, physical therapists are among the happiest with their careers. The job involves helping people, and it offers a financial reward as well. However, physical therapy is a challenging career. It can be demanding and complicated. As with all careers, it is best to learn as much as possible about it before making a final decision. Important considerations include the amount of education needed, varying jobs within the career, job requirements, and the future outlook of the profession.

chapter 1

WHAT IS A PHYSICAL THERAPIST?

Therapy is the treatment of a health problem. Many kinds of therapists focus on specific parts of the body. Some help people with mental disorders. Others help people with their speech. Physical therapists aid patients in moving, reducing pain, and restoring body function. They may work with a patient to prevent a disability as well. Some patients are born needing help with their bodies. Others become disabled later in life. All people experience differences in body function as they age.

Physical therapy has been around for thousands of years. As long as people have been promoting exercise for a healthy body or massage to soothe pain, there has been physical therapy. However, physical therapy as a profession is relatively new. During and after World War I (1914–1918), injured soldiers needed professionals to help them heal and return to their daily lives. At first, these people—usually women—were called reconstruction aides. They gave hope to soldiers who had lost limbs or suffered other severe wounds. The aides taught them how to become active again in spite of their disabilities.

In 1921, physical therapists formed their first professional association, the American Women's Physical Therapeutic Association. Led by president Mary McMillan, the association included 274 members. By the end of the 1930s, the

WHO'S SPECIALIZED

The first specialization education program, focusing on cardiopulmonary medicine, began in 1978. The American Physical Therapy Association (APTA) reports that as of 2008, 8,408 physical therapists have been certified as specialists. Almost five thousand of these are orthopedic PTs. The least common with a little more than one hundred specialists is cardiopulmonary physical therapy. The women's health specialization exam was first offered in 2009, making it the newest specialization certification.

association changed its name to the American Physiotherapy Association. Men were admitted, and membership grew to just under one thousand. After World War II (1939–1945), physical therapists not only worked with soldiers but also with the many children and adults who were suffering from the disease polio. Physical therapists proved that they were needed just as much as doctors.

The sudden rise of the physical therapy profession may stem from one of the main differences between PTs and doctors. Doctors work to locate a patient's problem and will then prescribe a treatment—which may include physical therapy. Usually, the doctor will continue to see the patient for a period of time to see if he or she has progressed. Unlike doctors, physical therapists work alongside a patient during his or her rehabilitation. They may see a patient every day or a few times a week. They can see if the treatment is working and, if not, make changes. PTs offer a commitment of progress and time that most doctors cannot in today's health care system.

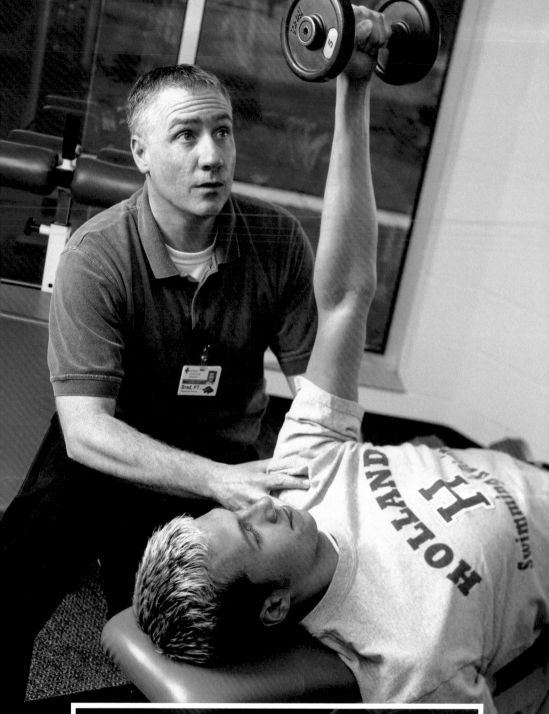

Sports medicine physical therapists may work in a variety of environments, including schools, general medical practices, or athletic facilities.

TYPES OF PHYSICAL THERAPY

Like doctors, physical therapists may practice general medicine, like a family doctor, or specialize in a certain kind of medicine, like a pediatrician. All PTs have some knowledge and experience in all areas of medicine. Physical therapists who choose to specialize are prepared to treat patients within that area of medicine. They study more about certain parts and functions of the body, as well as specific disorders, disabilities, and diseases. Below are the current areas of specialization in physical therapy according to the American Physical Therapy Association (APTA).

ORTHOPEDIC MEDICINE

Orthopedics is the branch of medicine that deals with bones, joints, ligaments, tendons, and muscles. These are the parts of the body that are necessary for movement. The largest number of specializing physical therapists focuses on orthopedics. Orthopedics is a basic part of most physical therapy plans. However, as a specialty, "ortho" PTs may help people with back pain, broken bones, hip and joint replacements, and arthritis.

SPORTS MEDICINE

Sports medicine focuses on injuries that happen to athletes on and off the field. Sports medicine PTs need to figure out a safe, effective, and speedy way to get an athlete back to his or her sport. They need to work toward prevention of injury and of re-injury as well. Athletic injuries may involve branches of medicine other than the more obvious orthopedic injuries; such injuries may be due to heart or lung problems. Often, a sports medicine PT needs to be a teacher to the athletes and

Research studies suggest that physical therapy can help reduce some symptoms of the neurological condition Alzheimer's disease.

help them understand how to protect their bodies. Some professional teams employ a physical therapist to work with their athletes. Even dance companies have PTs on staff.

NEUROLOGY

Neurology is the branch of medicine that deals with the structure and function of the nervous system. The brain, spinal cord, and a network of nerves are responsible for sending messages throughout the body to make movement possible. A disease or disorder of the nervous system can result in an inability to move or nonvoluntary movement. Some common neurological problems include stroke, brain injury, Alzheimer's disease, spinal cord injury, and cerebral palsy. PTs work with patients in balancing and walking.

CARDIOPULMONARY MEDICINE

Cardiovascular medicine involves the heart and blood vessels. Pulmonary medicine deals with the lungs. These areas are a combined physical therapy specialization. People who have had heart or lung surgery, or who suffer from diseases of the heart and lungs, may need rehabilitation with a physical therapist who is knowledgeable in these areas. Cardiopulmonary physical therapists help patients achieve the level of endurance and independence that they had prior to surgery and illness.

ELECTROPHYSIOLOGY

Electrophysiology is the study of the way electricity interacts with cells and tissues in the body. In other kinds of medical careers, electrophysiology focuses on correcting heart disorders, such as an irregular heartbeat. In physical therapy, electrical currents are used to reduce pain. The currents can prevent nerves from sending pain messages to the brain. Electricity can also be used to reduce inflammation, heal wounds, and keep blood flowing through muscles and limbs that a patient is unable to exercise.

PEDIATRIC MEDICINE

Pediatrics is the branch of medicine that concerns the care and development of children. Young patients may have the same problems as adults in all areas of medicine. Yet children need specific treatments, since their bodies are still developing. For example, many children don't have the ability or the necessary concentration to lift weights to build strength. The physical therapists assisting them may need to consider other methods of building strength, such as holding a ball. Pediatric PTs work to improve motor skills, balance, and endurance along with other bodily functions.

GERIATRIC MEDICINE

Geriatric physical therapists treat a number of different

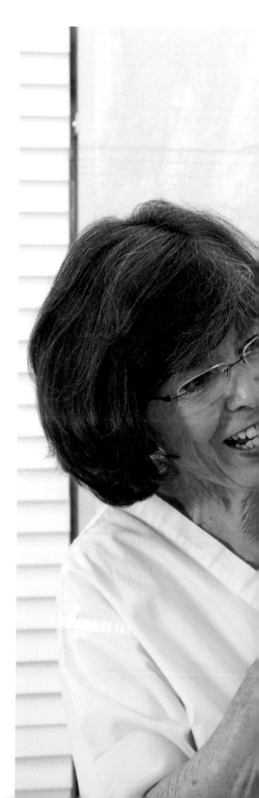

Geriatric PTs use their understanding of the physical changes that accompany the process of aging to plan programs of exercise for elderly patients.

problem areas in the body, but in older adults. As people age, they are more likely to experience arthritis, osteoporosis, cancer, Alzheimer's disease, and hip and joint replacement. An older patient may need a different treatment plan than a stronger, more able-bodied patient. For example, a patient with Alzheimer's disease may not be able to tell the physical therapist what is wrong or how a treatment is working. A geriatric PT must look for other signs to know how the patient is responding to a treatment.

WOMEN'S HEALTH

A physical therapist specializing in women's health focuses on women and their unique needs. Women struggling with pain, disorders, or disabilities may need therapy that is specially designed with their gender in mind. Pregnant women especially need special care to ensure that their growing baby is not harmed.

chapter 2

THE TREATMENT PLAN

The physical therapist functions as a coach. Just as a basketball coach needs to plan a strategy to win, a physical therapist needs to plan an appropriate treatment for his or her patient. This is one of the many reasons why physical therapists are so valuable. They recognize that each patient is unique and, therefore, needs a unique treatment.

When a patient first meets with a physical therapist, the PT will look at his or her medical history. It is important to know not only the patient's current ailment but also his or her past problems. A PT must be sure not to rehabilitate one area, only to harm another. Next, he or she tests the patient's strength. The physical therapist assigns a form of therapy that the patient will be able to handle. For example, if a geriatric patient needs to build strength in his or her arm, the PT must know how much the patient can lift.

The physical therapist also measures endurance. Can the patient do an exercise for a certain period of time? If a patient has lung disease, he or she may be able to take only a few steps before running out of breath. In that case, the PT will start the patient with small periods of exercise and then build up to longer periods. Similarly, the PT checks the patient's range of motion—how much the patient can move body parts. More tests include coordination, balance, posture, breathing, and motor skills.

Balance exercises are one facet of many fall-prevention programs for the elderly. This type of physical therapy can help patients avoid the need for rehabilitation therapy.

The PT determines if the patient is capable of living at home, or if he or she would be better off staying at a special facility during treatment. If the patient is in danger of further injury while living at home, the physical therapist will suggest an alternative setting for treatment.

After looking at all of these factors in the patient's life, the PT develops a treatment plan to help the patient's condition and achieve a standard of wellness. The plan may include a series of small goals in addition to the final goal. The plan includes strategies to reach the final goal. It also states a purpose for these strategies so that the patient and other health professionals understand why they are doing what they are doing—how the strategies lead to the goal.

The treatment plan to achieve the goal or goals may include one strategy or many. It may involve activities performed by a patient alone at home or under the watch of a physical therapist in an office. The treatment may last a few weeks or even years. Everything depends on the condition of the patient. As the treatment plan progresses, it may change. The physical therapist and the patient will talk about how the treatment is working. The following are some treatments that physical therapists use.

EXERCISES

Some injuries and illnesses should not be rehabilitated using exercise. However, a PT can plan an exercise routine if appropriate. People often think of exercise as active. However, in physical therapy, some exercise is passive; the PT moves the patient's body. Exercise can also be active-assisted, meaning the physical therapist and patient work together.

Physical therapists teach exercises that help build strength using weights. Other exercises simply use the weight of certain body parts. Strong muscles, joints, tendons, and ligaments also tend to have less aches, stiffness, pains, and injuries. To make the lungs and heart stronger, PTs design programs that work these organs. The heart is a muscle that can be trained like other muscles to regain strength. The lungs and the muscles around them need exercise, too. The exercises that a PT might recommend may involve walking or arm movements to increase the blood flow and breathing rate.

Many illnesses and open-chest surgeries, such as heart surgery, weaken the muscles of the chest. Some people lose their ability to cough, which is important to rid the body of disease. Physical therapists can help build these muscles to help people cough and breathe deeply.

The full amount of motion that can occur at a joint is called the range of motion (ROM). If the ROM at a joint is less than normal, there may be certain activities that cannot be performed. For example, if a patient's shoulder has a decreased ROM, that patient may not be able to reach an object that is above his or her head. In order to maintain normal ROM, joints must be moved quite often through their available range. PTs teach patients range-of-motion exercises.

Mobility Training

Many physical therapists work with patients so that they can return to activities that are a part of daily living. Exercises like the kinds that are listed above are one aspect of that. Another large part is achieving mobility. Many people lose some sense of balance as they get older, which can lead to injuries. Exercises that address balance include stretching, strengthening, and walking. PTs help geriatric patients with balance problems so that they don't stop exercising and completing the activities of daily living.

This patient is using a trampoline as part of her recovery program. She must work to stabilize her leg muscles while balancing on one leg at a time.

Gait is the name for all the different parts of walking. Gait training focuses on helping a person develop the easiest and most effective strategies for walking. Treatment involves preventing injuries and developing strategies to increase stability and speed.

Mobility aids are used to help people get to where they want to go. Some mobility aids are walkers, crutches, canes, and wheelchairs. PTs choose the best mobility aid for their patients and teach them how to use it. If the mobility aid is not used properly, it will not be as helpful as it should be and may even be harmful.

If patients lose a part of their body, they may use a prosthesis, or an artificial limb. A device that helps support a weakened muscle or joint is called an orthotic device. A leg brace is an orthotic device. PTs teach patients to move with prosthetic and orthotic devices. Often, balance and coordination exercises are involved in this type of training.

Manual Therapy

Manual therapy is one of the most widely used therapies. "Manual" means doing something with one's hands. Massage is perhaps the most well-known technique. It can accomplish several goals: pain reduction, muscle relaxation, and increased circulation. Massage is often used in conjunction with other therapies.

Some diseases, such as cystic fibrosis, may involve a buildup of mucus in the lungs. PTs can apply "percussions" and "vibrations" as a way to loosen it. Percussion is force applied to the chest using a cupped hand or device. The loosened mucus is then easier to cough out. Vibrations or patting the chest help move the mucus as well. People suffering from certain lung diseases might suffocate without these treatments.

ANCIENT PHYSICAL THERAPY

People may think that using electricity in medicine is a new idea. Surprisingly, this method of treatment goes back thousands of years. Roman doctors used electric eels to treat arthritis. Later, medieval doctors reported that magnets could cure depression, arthritis, and even baldness.

Joint mobilization involves a PT moving a patient's joints. The joints may feel tight, stiff, or painful. Loosening the joint can often relieve the pain. In order to prevent the pain from returning, other treatments need to be performed, such as stretching and strengthening exercises. There are many different movements of mobilization. Some decrease pain, and others help increase range of movement.

MODALITIES

Modalities are devices—some simple and some complex—that aid in physical therapy and exercise. Although the name sounds complex, people use modalities every day for pain relief. Heating pads and ice packs are modalities. Physical therapists use heat to relax muscles and improve blood circulation. Some heat packs may be as warm as 160 degrees Fahrenheit (71 degrees Celsius), so a professional is needed in their application. Cold therapy, also called cryotherapy, causes blood vessels to tighten. It can be helpful in reducing swelling.

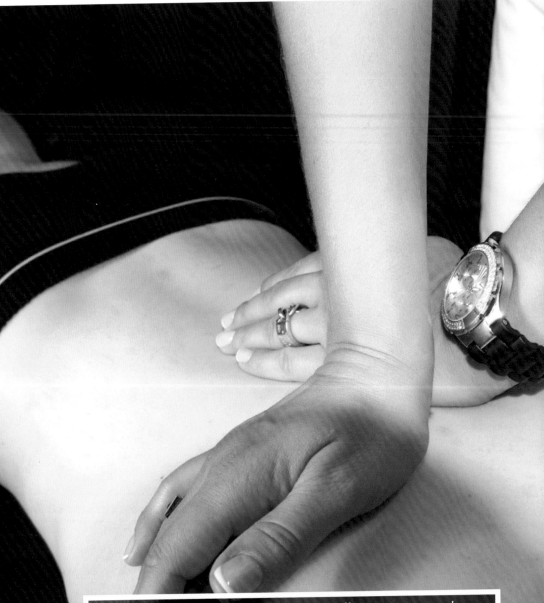

Massage is used to increase circulation as well as to warm muscles, tendons, and ligaments. Modalities such as electrotherapy can achieve similar effects.

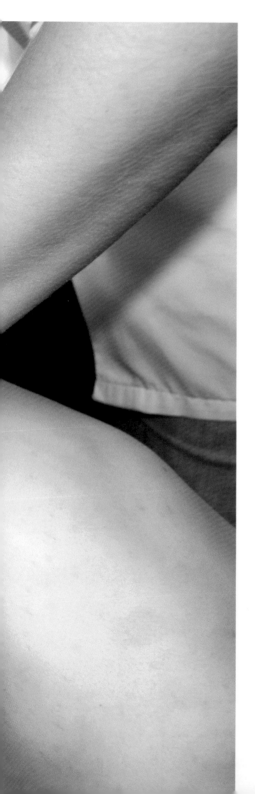

Ultrasound is another modality. Ultrasound devices create high-frequency sound waves that heat body tissues deep within the body. The heat increases flexibility and promotes healing.

Electrotherapy is the use of electrical currents to relieve muscles and nerves. The heat created brings blood to the tissue, which can speed the healing process. Coma and paralyzed patients cannot move their muscles voluntarily. In these cases, electricity may be used as a means to stimulate the patients' muscles in order to keep the blood flowing and to reduce muscle atrophy. Electricity can also be used to control pain. Tools called TENS (transcutaneous electrical nerve stimulation) units can be used by patients in their homes. PTs instruct patients how best to use these modalities.

Traction is a pulling force used to lessen pain and increase flexibility. PTs may use traction manually or using a device. Electric traction units create a pulling force through ropes, halters, and straps.

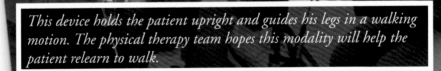

This device holds the patient upright and guides his legs in a walking motion. The physical therapy team hopes this modality will help the patient relearn to walk.

Water is another important part of physical therapy. Treatment using water is called hydrotherapy or aquatherapy. In such therapy, the water supports the body, and heated water decreases muscle stiffness and pain. Hydrotherapy programs, including whirlpools and heated pools, are used for people with many medical conditions, including arthritis and stroke. Water exercises are also prescribed as a cardiovascular exercise to improve overall fitness and health.

These are just some of the therapies available to PTs. Not only do physical therapists have to use their brains to construct treatment plans, they also have to use their bodies to guide patients through their programs. PTs need to be healthy and fit themselves, as their work with patients often involves exercise. They bend, crouch, lift, stand, swim, pull, push, walk, run, and support. Physical therapists definitely can't say they have a "desk job."

chapter 3

Becoming a
Physical Therapist

B
ecoming a physical therapist requires years of education. Even physical therapists choosing not to specialize need to understand the many systems of the human body and the ailments that affect them. The educational experience prepares PTs to be truly knowledgeable health care professionals. Young people who become PTs often agree that they enjoyed, and performed well in, high school science and health classes. For high school students, volunteering with the school athletic trainer is a good way to gain hands-on skills. Students of all ages can gain valuable experience volunteering at nursing homes, schools, and day care centers. A variety of volunteer opportunities can introduce future physical therapists to the many aspects of the career.

COLLEGE

Physical therapy programs require a degree from an accredited college or university. A few programs do combine the undergraduate and graduate degrees. However, physical therapy students should still expect to attend school for at least six years. An undergraduate degree requires classes from different subjects—a well-rounded education. Not only do graduates

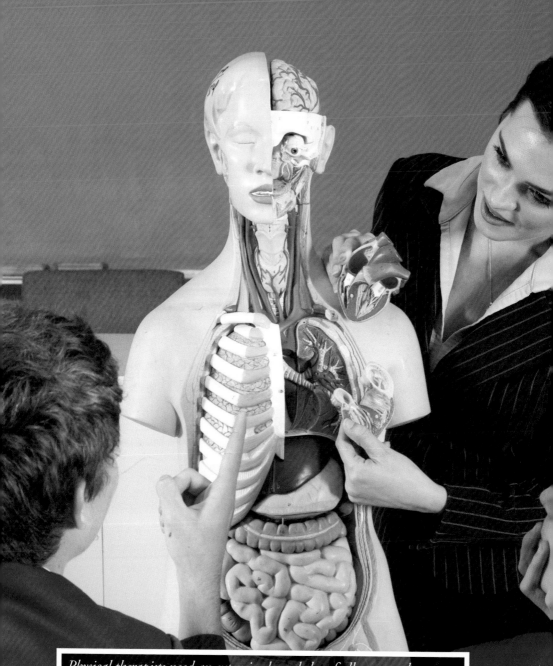

Physical therapists need an extensive knowledge of all parts and processes of the human body. Biology and other high school coursework can lay a good foundation for later studies.

know about science, but they can also read, write, and calculate. To enter a physical therapy program, the kind of undergraduate degree a student has matters less than the courses he or she took. Undergraduate students should complete courses in anatomy and physiology, biology, chemistry, psychology, statistics, mathematics, and physics. In addition, more than 75 percent of physical therapy programs require a minimum grade point average (GPA) of 3.0. College students should work with a counselor or adviser to make sure they complete the requirements of the physical therapy program they wish to pursue.

Before admitting a student, many physical therapy programs require volunteer experience in the physical therapy department of a hospital or clinic. Some schools require up to 150 hours of work related to physical therapy before the student can enter the program. They may also ask for letters of recommendation from teachers or physical therapists. Some

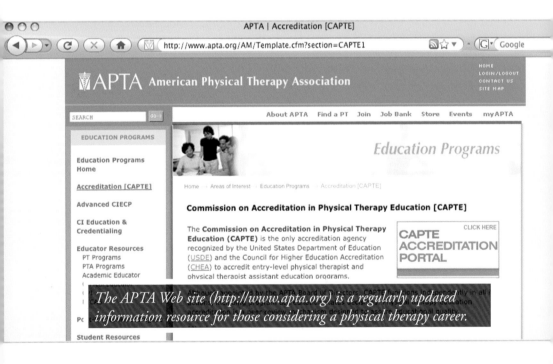

The APTA Web site (http://www.apta.org) is a regularly updated information resource for those considering a physical therapy career.

schools may require test scores from a graduate exam called the Graduate Record Examination, or GRE, as well.

CHOOSING A PHYSICAL THERAPY PROGRAM

There is much to consider when choosing a physical therapy school. The most important factor is the school's accreditation. The physical therapy program must have accreditation by the Commission on Accreditation in Physical Therapy Education (CAPTE). CAPTE is the national organization that reviews each school so that its physical therapy program offers the appropriate courses and a high-quality education. According to the APTA, there are more than two hundred accredited physical therapist education programs in the United States.

To help students apply to more than one program at a time, the APTA provides an online application process called the Physical Therapist Centralized Application Service (PTCAS). The PTCAS makes it possible for a single application to be sent to multiple physical therapist education programs. Applications can be quite lengthy and complicated. PTCAS has made the application process much easier.

Other considerations for choosing a physical therapy program include:

- Distance from home
- Class size
- Cost and available financial aid and scholarships
- Success of past students in passing the license exam
- Success of graduates in getting jobs
- Experience and reputation of teachers
- Student activities and organizations
- Opportunities to practice physical therapy in school
- Doctoral and other available professional programs

Professional Organizations

Joining professional organizations, even while in school, has many benefits. Organizations can provide information about future jobs. Another advantage of membership is learning about new research and practices in physical therapy. The American Physical Therapy Association is perhaps the most important of these professional organizations for U.S. physical therapists. Members are presented job opportunities, classes and lectures, and places to meet other physical therapists. Besides the APTA, physical therapists may want to join their state physical therapy organization as well as more local groups. Meetings and information for these groups may focus on community issues.

Besides finding out these answers online and through school tours and materials, past and current students of the program are good resources. They can offer valuable and honest information about their experiences.

A degree program in physical therapy usually lasts two years. It starts with basic science courses, such as biology, chemistry, and physics. It then becomes more in-depth about the human body and development, disease, disorders, and therapies. Besides learning in a classroom, students complete internships, called clinicals, in hospitals, clinics, and other settings. They are supervised and taught how to apply their classroom knowledge to real-life situations.

Changes are happening within physical therapy education in the United States. In the past, students graduated from college with an undergraduate degree in physical therapy. Now this is impossible. Several years ago, a physical therapist would complete his or her education program with a master's degree. Now most accredited physical therapist programs are offering doctoral degrees. The APTA's aim is that the majority of practicing physical therapists will possess a doctoral degree in the future. Many schools offer a "transitional" doctoral degree for those wishing to return to school to attain this higher degree. Doctoral degrees are called "clinical" doctorates. This means PTs use them in their work or to teach in a physical therapist education program.

THE NATIONAL EXAM

After completing a degree in physical therapy, PTs need to pass at least one more test before they can practice. This test is called the National Physical Therapy Exam (NPTE). It's taken on a computer, and it consists of 250 multiple-choice questions. The exam taker has five hours to complete the test. The NPTE is graded on a scale from two hundred to eight hundred. A score of six hundred is passing. If the test-taker does not pass the NPTE, he or she can take the exam again. There are a number of resources available to prepare people for the test. The Federation of State Boards of Physical Therapy develops and administers the NPTE. Below are sample NPTE questions found on the federation's Web site:

1. After sitting at a computer station for two to three hours, an individual reports experiencing a sharp, localized pain in the left arm. When asked to show the location of the pain, the individual points to the area of the insertion of the deltoid. The pain disappears when the individual stands up and walks around briefly. Which of the following interventions is MOST likely to correct the problem?

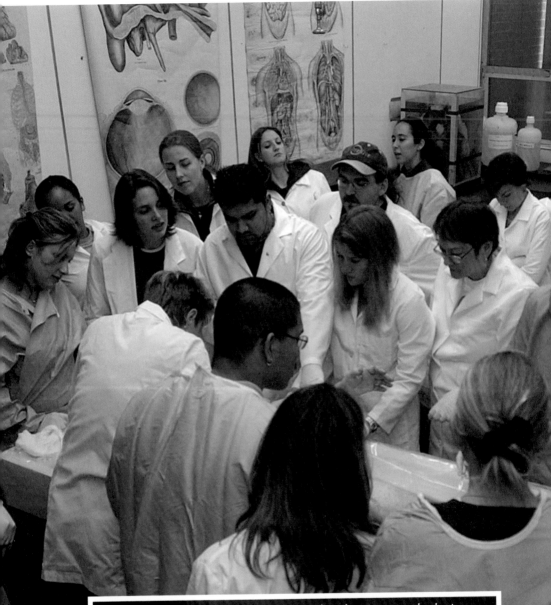

Anatomy classes may use a cadaver, as this class is, to study the inner workings of the human body. This practical experience allows students to apply their book knowledge to a real-life experience.

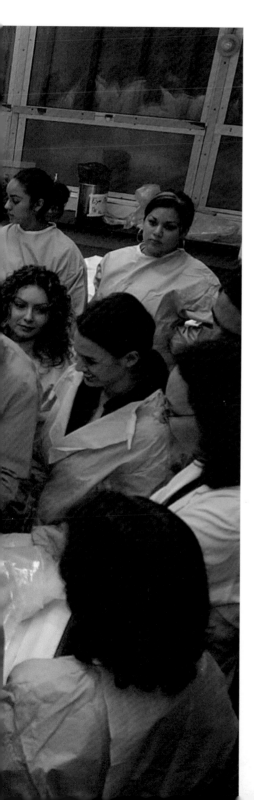

a. Isometric strengthening of the deltoid
b. Lumbar extension exercises in prone
c. Instruction in correct postural alignment in sitting
d. Instruction in shoulder active range of motion exercises

2. A patient with a medullary level vascular lesion has increased vagal nerve activity. Which of the following descriptions BEST represents the cardiovascular effects that occur when the patient transitions from supine to standing?

a. Rise in blood pressure and no change in heart rate
b. Drop in blood pressure and no change in heart rate
c. Rise in blood pressure and an increase in heart rate
d. Drop in blood pressure and an increase in heart rate

Answers: 1. c; 2. b

The passing rate for NPTE test-takers who have completed an accredited program in the

United States is more than 80 percent. This evidence suggests that most test-takers are well prepared after their classroom and clinical experiences.

BEYOND THE EXAM

The NPTE score is sent to the applicant's state licensing board. This organization is responsible for granting licenses to PTs. Each state licensing board has a set of requirements for the applicant to fulfill. The state license helps employers and patients to know that the PT has been tested and found to be competent.

For example, the New York State licensing board requires at least a master's degree in physical therapy from an accredited program and a passing score on the NPTE. A fee must be submitted with a form requesting a license as well. In addition, a license requires that the candidate "be of good moral character."

DEGREE INITIALS

After becoming a physical therapist, a person has the letters "PT" added after his or her name. Following that, more initials tell others about the additional degrees and certifications that a physical therapist has. "MPT" means master's degree in physical therapy. "DPT" means doctor of physical therapy. "CCS" is cardiovascular and pulmonary certified specialist. "ECS" is clinical electro-physiologic certified specialist. "GCS" is geriatric certified specialist. "NCS" is neurologic certified specialist. "OCS" is orthopedic certified specialist. "PCS" is pediatric certified specialist. "SCS" is sports certified specialist. And "WHCS" is women's health certified specialist.

Many states and job sites require a police background check for any criminal activities in a PT's past.

Some states require additional exams. Students who studied in other countries or whose first language is not English may be required to prove their language skills and knowledge. They can find the procedure to follow through their state licensing board.

After receiving a license to practice, physical therapists can enter the working world. Some may wish to specialize in one of the areas described in chapter 1. In order to take a specialization exam, the candidate must have a license and more than

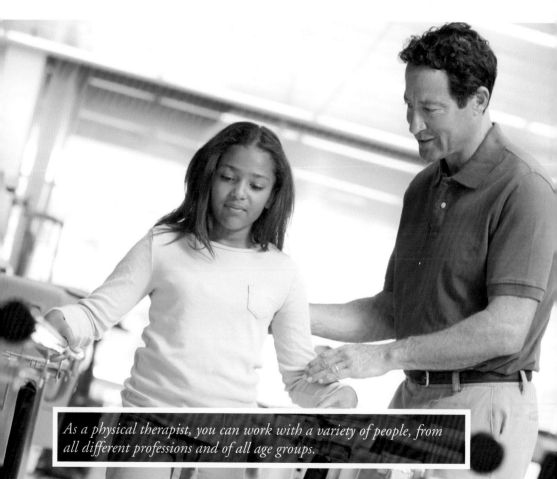

As a physical therapist, you can work with a variety of people, from all different professions and of all age groups.

two thousand hours of experience working in that specific area of medicine. A test is available for each certification. Upon passing the test, physical therapists are granted a specialization certification. They must retake the test every ten years.

ALWAYS STUDENTS

Physical therapists are expected to continue learning by participating in classes and workshops. These continuing education courses are measured in continuing education units (CEUs). Each state licensing board requires a physical therapist to earn a certain number of CEUs in order to keep his or her license. For example, in South Carolina, one CEU is described as ten "contact hours" in an organized educational opportunity. A physical therapist in that state must complete three CEUs every two years, or thirty hours of education. This requirement keeps PTs educated about the best options and methods of care for their patients.

chapter 4

STARTING A CAREER

Before physical therapists complete their education, they will have gone through clinical training in a variety of settings, including hospitals, nursing homes, clinics, and schools. According to the U.S. Bureau of Labor Statistics, about six out of ten physical therapists work in hospitals or clinics. Most of the remaining physical therapists travel to people's homes or work in nursing homes, doctors' offices, schools, and sports and fitness clubs. Wherever they choose, most PTs can expect to work a forty-hour week, which may include evenings and weekends. After graduation and licensure, physical therapists have to make the choice: where do they want to work?

CHOOSING A WORKPLACE

One factor in choosing a first job site is the specialization or area of interest. For instance, a physical therapist wishing to specialize in electrophysiology should not practice in a school. A PT interested in practicing many forms of therapy should not work in a cardiopulmonary clinic. There also may be different job titles and responsibilities for physical therapists within each setting. For example, a group of physical therapists within a hospital may have a physical therapy director who oversees their work. In a smaller clinic, a PT may be the sole therapist. Here is a look at places where physical therapists can find work.

HOSPITALS

Physical therapists can encounter a variety of patients in a hospital setting. Some PTs may work only in certain sections of the hospital. Others may work in many. A common patient problem in a hospital is loss of strength from long periods of

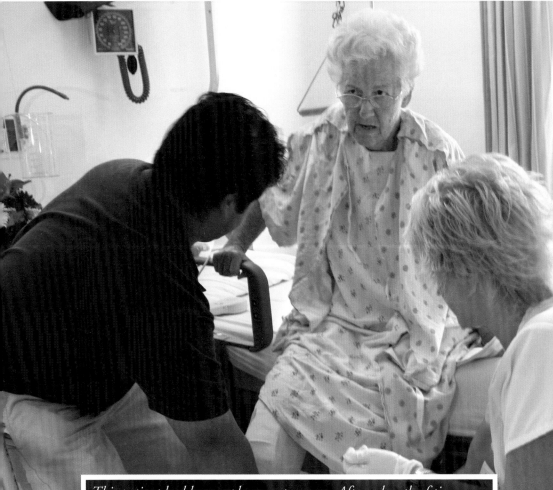

This patient had knee-replacement surgery. After a length of time resting, she needs to begin the process of regaining her mobility at a rehabilitation hospital.

time in bed. A physical therapist can teach this patient how to regain strength and mobility. Burn victims need physical therapy, including active and passive exercise. People with burns suffer pain, itching, and anxiety both from the burn and the healing of wounds. Some studies suggest that massage helps ease these symptoms. Physical therapy can improve movement and function in the burn area and reduce scarring. People in a coma require physical therapy, too. The PT will move and stimulate the patient's limbs until the patient can do so independently.

The duties of PTs in a hospital are as varied as the problems of the patients in the hospital. However, the goal remains getting the patient fit to return home. A 2007 Wake Forest Medical University study showed that the use of physical therapy in hospital intensive care units (ICUs) reduced the amount of time a patient remained in the ICU.

REHABILITATION HOSPITALS

Sometimes patients need a long period of time to recover from an injury or surgery. They may be sent to a rehabilitation hospital or center. Physical therapists work with these patients until they are able to go home. Patients in rehabilitation centers are often those with severe injuries or conditions, such as spinal cord injuries, strokes, and chronic pain. Some of these people need to learn the simplest of movements. People who lose their limbs through accidents, diabetes, or circulation problems need PTs. They may need to learn to walk with or without the use of orthotics and prosthetics. PTs in a rehabilitation hospital must work to keep the patient optimistic about recovery.

CLINICS AND OFFICES

Unlike hospitals and rehabilitation centers, clinics provide treatment for patients who can live at home. Clinics that provide these services are called outpatient clinics. They may be associated with a hospital or be privately owned. They may treat a variety of problems or specialize in one area, such as pain management. Some clinics specialize in physical therapy. Patients seeking help at a physical therapy clinic may be suffering from back, neck, or other limb pain; need after-surgery rehabilitation; and need help caring for wounds. Physical therapists can provide multiple treatment sessions through an outpatient clinic. Doctors' offices often hire PTs to provide treatment as well.

NURSING HOMES AND ASSISTED-LIVING FACILITIES

Nursing home PTs practice geriatric medicine. They must keep the elderly patients moving to prevent muscle atrophy. Older patients need to keep exercising to keep their bodies healthy enough for the activities of daily living, such as bathing, eating, and dressing. They may need to learn how to do these things while using a wheelchair or walker. Physical therapists in nursing homes must also aid in easing conditions that afflict the elderly, such as Alzheimer's disease, osteoporosis, and Parkinson's disease. Nursing homes are sometimes called assisted-living facilities. They aren't only for the elderly. Some younger people who cannot live at home unassisted must live in assisted-living facilities to receive care.

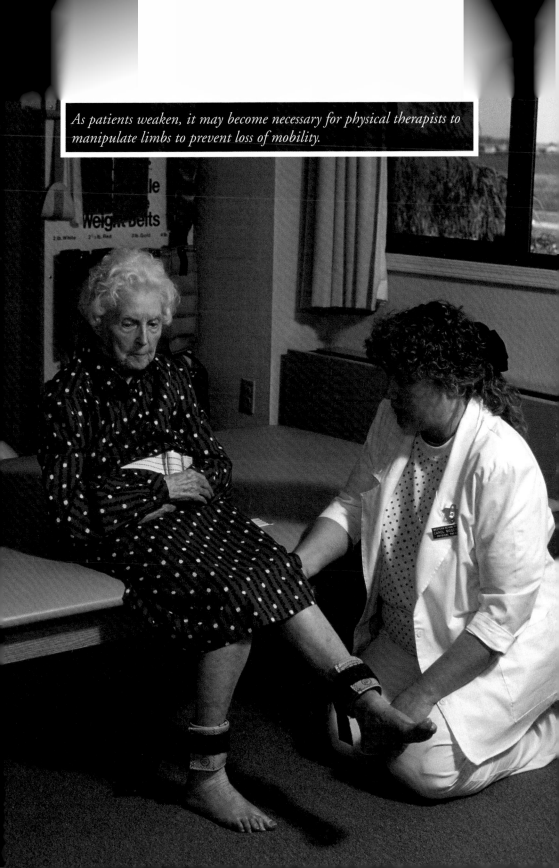

As patients weaken, it may become necessary for physical therapists to manipulate limbs to prevent loss of mobility.

SCHOOLS

Many schools hire physical therapists to work with children who need rehabilitation in order to fully participate in school. School-based physical therapy focuses on a child's ability to move independently in a school. The PT helps the student walk around the classroom and take part in activities to make his or her school experience as normal as possible. PTs for each student are on a team that includes teachers, parents, and other therapists. Physical therapists in schools may have special knowledge of pediatric medicine in order to best care for kids.

PRIVATE HOMES

At times, a patient cannot travel to a clinic for regular physical therapy treatments. In that case, the patient needs a PT who makes home visits. Agencies specializing in home health care send physical therapists to people's homes. It can be a great advantage for patients to have physical therapy at home. For example, the PT can see how far the patient needs to walk from the bedroom to the kitchen. He or she can see how many steps are in the house, and so on.

SELF-EMPLOYMENT

Some physical therapists choose to be self-employed. They have their own practice, find their own clients, and may do work with doctors' offices, home health care agencies, or other medical facilities. Self-employed physical therapists can set their own hours and enjoy being their own boss.

WRITING A RÉSUMÉ

After choosing a place to work, physical therapists need to start the job hunt. Just as they applied to school, they need to apply for a job position. The education process gives PTs a lot of experience to present to possible employers. However, physical therapists need to know how to make themselves stand out. Many other job candidates are just starting out or have years of experience behind them. Beginning a career is not as simple as writing a résumé, a list of the job candidate's accomplishments. However, a résumé—sometimes called a curriculum vitae—is the first necessary step. It gives the employer a "snapshot" of the physical therapist before meeting him or her. Résumés may look different for different jobs. A sample PT résumé on the APTA's Web site includes the following information:

- Name, address, and contact information
- College, graduate school, and advanced degrees
- Licenses
- Detailed lists of professional experience relating to physical therapy
- Continuing education and professional development classes
- Teaching activities, including presentations and clinical education
- Publications in books, medical magazines, and journals
- Research activities
- Professional society and organization memberships
- Honors and awards received
- Any other notable skills, such as knowledge of foreign languages or computers

If possible, job candidates should personally deliver their résumés to the office, unless other directions are given. They might be able to make a good first impression on their future employer. It also shows an eagerness for the job. Next, the employer chooses a number of people to meet for a face-to-face interview. The candidates need to know how best to present themselves.

Going for the Interview

Being interviewed for a job can make some people nervous. After all, they are being judged by their words and actions. However, an interview shows that the employer is already impressed with the candidate's résumé. Now the employer wants to see how the candidate acts in person. The following interview tips can apply to any job opportunity:

- Arrive early, perhaps ten to fifteen minutes early.
- Bring an extra résumé.
- Act like a coworker with whom the employer would want to work. Be upbeat. Dress appropriately. Make eye contact.
- Be confident without bragging. Be honest about accomplishments. Do not talk too much or too little.
- State strengths that stand out among other PTs. Practice in front of a mirror. Verbal pauses such as "ums" and "ahs" can make a candidate seem unprepared.
- Be ready with good references. These should be professionals that can speak about your character and abilities.
- Write a thank-you note after the interview. It will remind the interviewer of you, one of possibly many. It shows thoughtfulness and courtesy.

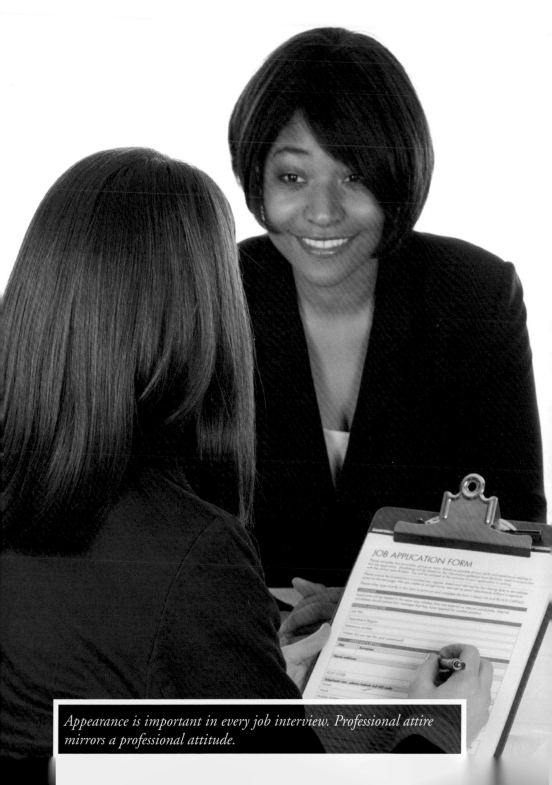

Appearance is important in every job interview. Professional attire mirrors a professional attitude.

ALTERNATIVE PHYSICAL THERAPY CAREERS

There are alternative ways to work within this career. Some physical therapists may choose to teach within a physical

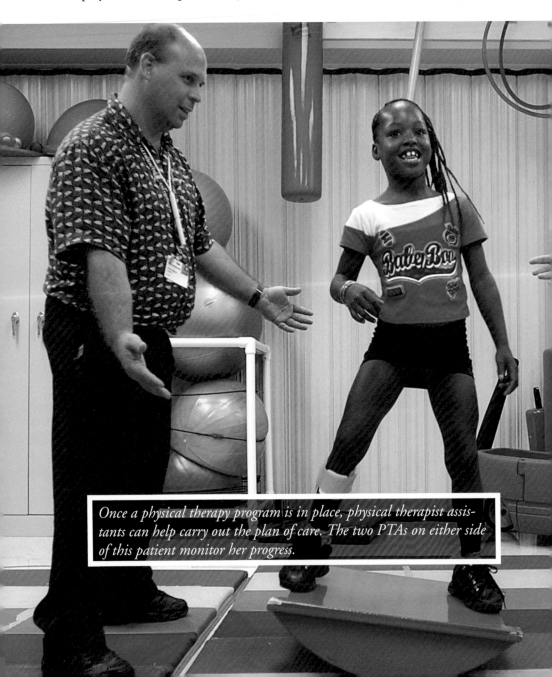

Once a physical therapy program is in place, physical therapist assistants can help carry out the plan of care. The two PTAs on either side of this patient monitor her progress.

therapy program rather than practice. They may instruct in a classroom or supervise students in clinicals. There are special degree programs offered for clinical instructors. Other PTs become medical researchers, studying new and accepted methods of therapy, and seeking better ways to improve quality of life for patients. However, some people who are interested in a career in physical therapy may find that they do not have the resources to attend a physical therapy education program. These people still have career options.

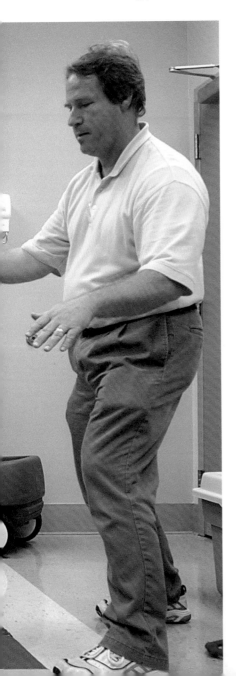

PHYSICAL THERAPIST ASSISTANTS

Physical therapist assistants, or PTAs, work under the direction of a physical therapist. Unlike PTs, PTAs do not examine patients, create a plan of care for them, or decide if they are fully rehabilitated. However, PTAs can guide patients through a treatment plan, collect data on their progress, and report their response to treatment. Physical therapist assistant programs can be found at universities, community colleges, and technical colleges. PTAs graduate from a two-year accredited program with an associate's degree. Different states have different rules about whether a physical therapist assistant needs a license or not. The Federation of State Boards of Physical Therapy collects information needed for PTAs in each state. PTAs generally have a lower salary than PTs.

PHYSICAL THERAPIST AIDES

Physical therapist aides work under PTs and PTAs. They are responsible for keeping treatment areas clean and ready for patient use. A physical therapist aide may also help patients move around in wheelchairs or support them in moving in other ways. In larger work settings, physical therapist aides may also do office work, such as keeping records and answering phones. Generally, physical therapist aides do not need as much medical knowledge as PTs or PTAs. They are not required to have a degree, and they earn less than PTAs. People who are interested in gaining valuable experience in physical therapy should consider becoming a physical therapist aide first.

chapter 5

CHALLENGES
AND REWARDS

P hysical therapists encounter all of the highs and lows
that accompany a career in health care. Words used
to describe a career in physical therapy can seem to
contradict each other: demanding, rewarding, drain-
ing, inspiring. A PT can experience all of these feelings on a
single day. Perhaps it is this variety that draws many physical
therapists to their work. Most still believe it is the best profession for them.

A group of physical therapists was asked in a survey for
U.S. News and World Report to describe their overall thoughts
about their job. More than three-quarters said they were
"very satisfied." Only clergy reported more glowing praise
of their occupation. Among the reasons given for the good
review were:

- Working face-to-face with people
- Seeing a patient progress toward wellness
- Spending time with patients
- Making decisions and often acting as your own boss
- Encountering a variety of situations, keeping work
  interesting
- Choosing to work normal work hours in most
  situations

- Wide variety of workplaces, from hospitals to private homes
- Positive outlook of the future job market

Most physical therapy patients feel they are satisfied as well. According to an APTA survey, 88 percent of physical

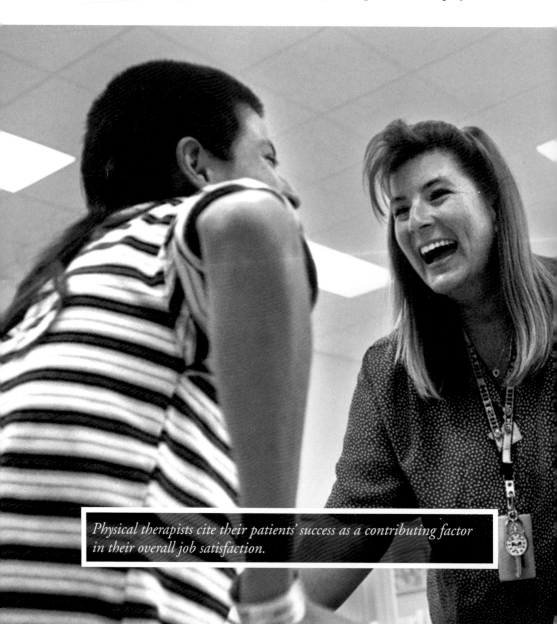

Physical therapists cite their patients' success as a contributing factor in their overall job satisfaction.

therapy patients reported that the care they received helped them return to normal activity, increased their range of motion, and relieved their pain. Eighty-four percent recommended their PT to someone else.

WHAT ABOUT SALARY?

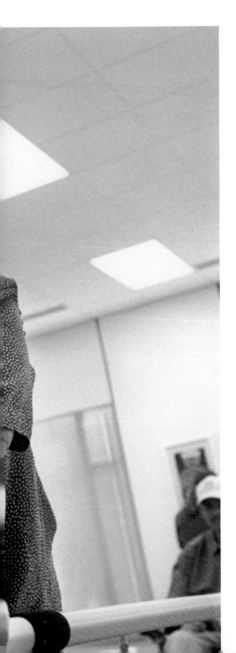

Although salary wasn't mentioned specifically in the above survey, it is another benefit of a PT's career. Salary depends on many factors. Within an organization, there may be different positions of authority and ranking. Another salary consideration is the experience of the PT. A physical therapist just hired from graduate school will likely earn less than a PT with ten years of experience. Another aspect is location. There are often job rewards for places that need physical therapists. The kind of place where the PT chooses to work is another salary factor.

According to the APTA, more than 172,000 physical therapists are licensed in the United States today. The highest 10 percent of PTs earn more than $86,000. The U.S. Bureau of Labor Statistics Web site maintains up-to-date salary information, including how job site and specialization impact earnings.

PHYSICAL THERAPISTS IN THE MILITARY

The roots of modern physical therapy are in the military. Physical therapists still serve an important role in the armed services today. They help injured service members recover. They may work with long-term injuries as well, helping people live a normal life. They also work to prevent injuries. Physical therapists who serve in the military may work in their home countries or overseas. They may be employed in hospitals, clinics, or military stations. They may work on shore or on a boat. They are called to treat all kinds of ailments and, therefore, remain an essential part of the armed services.

THE OTHER SIDE OF THE COIN

Like those working in any other career field, physical therapists have job criticisms, too, which they expressed in the *U.S. News and World Report* survey. Some criticisms naturally follow parts of the job that PTs admired. For instance, some love the energetic work environment, while others find it too physically demanding. After helping patients exercise all day, physical therapists may feel exercise fatigue themselves. While physical therapists love to see their patients reach their goals, they will also see some patients lose hope, fail, and even die. Sometimes the challenge of finding a cause of pain can be too difficult. At times, a patient may not be able to tell the PT. This, too, takes a toll on physical therapists.

The extensive education of physical therapists can prepare them well for the workplace. However, it can involve a lot of time and money. After graduation, PTs need to keep their licenses in good standing through continuing education units. These, too, can cost money and time. In addition, many physical therapists are finding that job candidates with doctorates are gaining a better foothold in the job market. In the future, more PTs may need to reach that level of education.

Another difficult factor in a physical therapist's day can be paperwork. Today's health care system involves a lot of contact with health insurance agencies. Careful records of the treatment process need to be kept. Also, patients cannot always pay for the amount of treatment that they need. At times, their insurance companies may refuse to cover their treatment altogether. These present very frustrating obstacles in a PT's life.

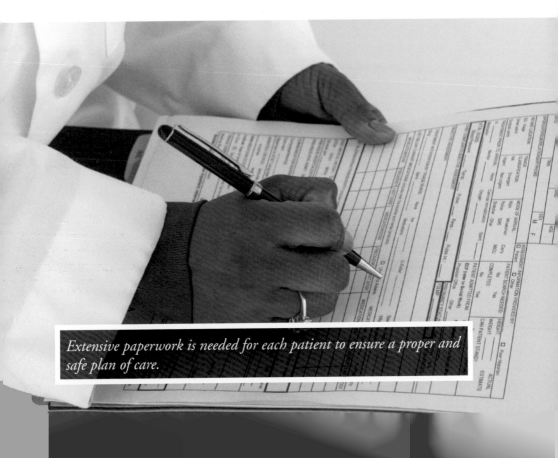

Extensive paperwork is needed for each patient to ensure a proper and safe plan of care.

A DAY IN THE LIFE

To know what a profession is really like, ask someone who's in it. He or she will likely offer some advice and insight that can't be taught in school. Kelly C. is a physical therapist in Connecticut. In this section, she offers some views of her life as a school-based physical therapist, as well as her thoughts about the challenges and rewards of her career.

WHERE DO YOU WORK?

I currently work in two school districts at several different schools for a total of eight schools per week. I have this type of arrangement because each district needed only a part-time PT. There isn't a huge need for PTs in schools. There is a greater need for occupational therapists and speech therapists. I have several schools because there are usually not enough children at a school to fill a day's worth of treatment. As you might imagine, scheduling can be tricky.

MEETING A MENTOR

New physical therapists and physical therapy students who are interested in knowing all sides of the profession may want an experienced mentor. The APTA provides the Member Mentoring Members (MMM) program. The program matches mentors with those seeking mentors. It is a free resource for the APTA members who are students, new professionals, and experienced professionals. Mentors can help with career, clinical, and professional issues. There is also a student-to-student group called Student Mentoring: Achieving & Reaching Together (SMART). More information is available on the APTA Web site.

WHAT CHALLENGES DO YOU FACE?

It's a great challenge to work around the student's class schedules. This is perhaps one of the hardest things about this type of setting. There is also not much space in a school to work. I don't have all the equipment available in a hospital or clinic, so I have to be creative and original.

The most difficult part of being a school-based PT is probably trying to decide what the child needs as a student, as opposed to what the child needs as a child. School-based therapy is meant to help the child benefit from their education. This means, for example, getting around the school, sitting for desk activities, and participating in physical education and recess. They may have difficulties that do not necessarily affect their education. As a professional trained to help reduce, prevent, and rehabilitate physical disabilities, I feel at times that I have to stop before I would like.

WITH WHOM DO YOU WORK?

I work alongside teachers, but also other health care professionals, namely occupational therapists, speech therapists, nurses, social workers, and psychologists. I occasionally speak with a doctor, but this is usually my request. This can be another challenge—making contact with a doctor despite both of our hectic schedules.

HOW DID YOU DECIDE TO WORK IN SCHOOLS?

I used to work in an adult rehabilitation center with people who suffered strokes, head injuries, spinal cord injuries, and other medical issues. I found the amount of tasks—scheduling, paperwork, billing, ordering equipment, treatment, and

OCCUPATIONAL THERAPISTS

Occupational therapy is the profession most directly responsible for addressing problems with fine motor skills and coordination. Occupational therapists (OTs) and physical therapists often work closely together. The OT helps with activities of daily living (ADL), such as dressing, eating, and household and workplace activities. They often focus on the use of hands and arms. In school settings, OTs may be asked to assist students with handwriting difficulties. More than PTs, OTs use psychology when working with their patients. Occupational therapists have a unique therapeutic approach to helping children manage their five senses within their environment.

meetings—made it difficult to get everything done in a day's work. This is what prompted me to leave that job and look toward the schools.

WHAT IS THE BEST PART OF BEING A PT?

The best part of being a PT is seeing someone improve their life because of the help that I've provided. This improvement may be allowing them to do something they couldn't before, providing a piece of equipment that makes life easier, or even offering information about how to get additional support.

PT is also a nice blend of medicine—everything from orthopedics, optometry, cardiopulmonary, pharmacology, etc. Someone who enjoys medicine and problem solving will find it to be a great profession. No two patients are alike, so it never gets boring.

HOW DID YOU KNOW YOU WANTED TO BE A PT?

I knew I wanted to study physical therapy when I was applying to colleges. I had been an athlete through high school and had needed physical therapy myself. I was really interested in the posters they had on the walls of all the bones and muscles.

DO YOU HAVE ANY SUGGESTIONS FOR FUTURE PTS?

One strong suggestion I have for anyone thinking about being a PT is to spend time with a PT, preferably in a variety of settings. Prior to college, I was only aware of the sports medicine part of physical therapy—and only a small part of that. The physical therapy program was difficult for me because I didn't have any experience. Students should talk with practicing PTs, volunteer in clinics and hospitals, or set up days to shadow a PT. The education is difficult and requires many years. You don't want to find out it's not what you really wanted. The more experiences someone has, the better off they may be. They may also encounter similar professions that appeal to them.

BABIES

Babies born early, or prematurely, need physical therapy as well. Forty weeks is the normal length for pregnancy. Babies born earlier than that can suffer a number of problems, including physical disability, hearing loss, blindness, and chronic diseases like asthma. According to the National Center for Health Statistics, about 12.8 percent of all babies are born premature. This number has risen in the past twenty years. Modern medicine is helping more babies survive than ever before, including newborns with severe medical issues. Future PTs will help these children live fuller and longer lives.

CHANGE IN GEOGRAPHY

Some physical therapists will need to relocate to treat patients. Populations in and around cities have been increasing, while populations in rural areas have been decreasing. Also, there has been a general movement of populations to the southern and western regions of the United States. While more PTs will be needed to

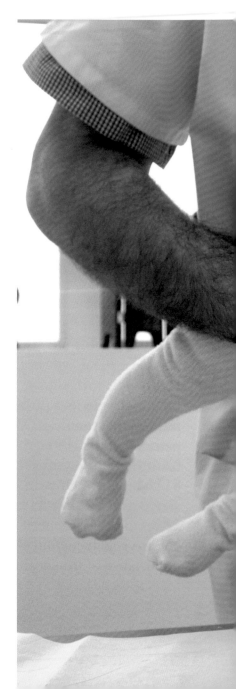

serve more populated areas, some will still be needed to care for patients in less populated areas. Higher salaries may be offered to physical therapists willing to relocate to rural areas to practice.

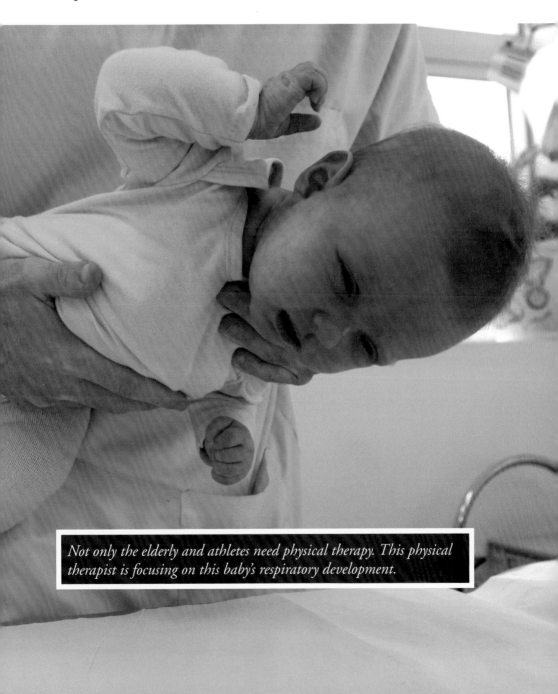

Not only the elderly and athletes need physical therapy. This physical therapist is focusing on this baby's respiratory development.

NEW TREATMENTS

Physical therapists will continue to develop new treatments and methods, expanding the range of physical therapy practices. In

For thousands of years, acupuncture has been practiced in Asia to relieve pain and promote an overall wellness in the body.

addition, growth may result from medical advances that allow for the survival of people with disabling conditions that were untreatable or fatal in the past.

PTs are also finding that more people are interested in

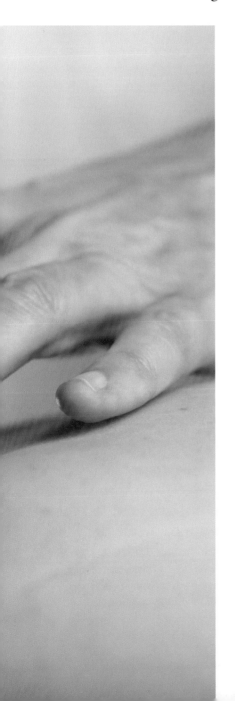

trying therapies like yoga and acupuncture. In fact, acupuncture, the method of inserting needles into the skin to treat disorders, is an accepted part of physical therapy in Canada. Many patients are interested in exploring options outside of drugs and prescription medicine, which can have harmful side effects, to treat their aches and pains.

Physical therapists do not offer quick fixes or magic pills. What they offer may be better. According to the APTA, physical therapists offer just two services: healing and caring. These services cover quite a lot. However, they tell us exactly what we need to know about physical therapy as a career.

HEALING, CARING, AND OTHER "MUST-HAVES"

Healing concerns a person's physical well-being. A substantial portion

ERGONOMICS

Ergonomics is the study of how workplace equipment can be used in safe, comfortable, and productive ways. Physical therapists use ergonomics when teaching people to prevent or recover from conditions like carpal tunnel syndrome and neck and back pain. These conditions are common to people who work long hours sitting at a computer. If left untreated, some of these ailments can become so severe that they lead to more disabling conditions. Many companies are employing PTs to prevent on-the-job injuries with ergonomics.

of this book has focused on the methods of healing that a PT uses. Healing therapies can be simple or complex. Caring, though, is more difficult to teach. Caring is concern for a patient's emotional well-being. It means connecting with a patient on a personal level. Emotional and mental health affects healing. Is the patient suffering from stress? Does the patient have the support he or she needs to successfully complete difficult exercises? These are some questions that a physical therapist may ask.

Caring is an aspect of the job that cannot be taught or learned. However, it is a "must-have" in a physical therapy career. Physical therapists must have strong "people skills" so that they can better teach patients how to care for themselves. After all, a PT cannot be with the patient all the time. In addition, physical therapists need to be able to communicate with patients' families. Medical care can be a hardship for patients and families alike. It helps when patients feel they can place their trust in a professional who will not only treat them but care for them as well.

The best advice for aspiring physical therapists is to keep reading, researching, and volunteering. These three activities will ensure that future PTs know what is expected of them and what they can expect to encounter in their future career. Within the career itself, there are countless paths to choose. This is both intimidating and exciting, but many things worth pursuing are. However, students who have fully prepared themselves before beginning a physical therapy career will find it a rewarding and satisfying opportunity to enrich people's lives in so many ways.

glossary

accreditation An official recognition for having met a standard.

ailment An illness or injury.

Alzheimer's disease An illness that causes mental problems, such as extreme forgetfulness.

anatomy The physical structure, especially internal, of a plant or animal.

arthritis An illness that causes swelling of the joints, stiffness, and pain.

atrophy Weakening or lessening in ability.

carpal tunnel syndrome A condition of pain or weakness in a hand or wrist caused by repetitive movements.

cerebral palsy A condition caused by brain damage at birth marked by a lack of muscle control.

chronic Lasting a long time or occurring often.

coordination Movement of body parts at the same time.

cystic fibrosis A disease that results in thick mucus blocking air passages.

diabetes A disorder that causes the body to produce an excessive amount of urine.

doctoral Relating to the highest degree offered by a university.

evaluate To examine something in order to judge its condition.

geriatric Relating to the elderly.

inflammation Swelling, redness, heat, and pain in an area of the body as a result of injury or infection.

ligament Tissue in the body that connects bones at a joint or supports another body part.

massage A treatment that involves rubbing or kneading the muscles.

mentor A trusted guide or teacher.

motor skill A function that involves precise movement of muscles with the intent to perform a specific act.

osteoporosis A disease in which bones become brittle and break easily.

passive Not actively participating.

physiology A branch of biology that deals with how living things function.

polio A severe infection that inflames the brain stem and spinal cord, sometimes leading to paralysis.

posture The way a person carries his or her body.

rehabilitation The process of making someone healthy again.

statistics The branch of math that deals with interpreting data.

tendon A cord of tissue that attaches a muscle to a bone or other body part.

American Physical Therapy Association
1111 North Fairfax Street
Alexandria, VA 22314-1488
(800) 999-2782
Web site: http://www.apta.org
The APTA is a national organization that works to advance
    physical therapy practice, research, and education.

Canadian Physiotherapy Association
2345 Yonge Street, Suite 410
Toronto, ON M4P 2E5
Canada
(800) 387-8679
Web site: http://www.physiotherapy.ca
This is a Canadian organization of physical therapists that
    provides resources and research for therapists and patients.

Federation of State Boards of Physical Therapy
124 West Street South
Alexandria, VA 22314
(703) 299-3100
Web site: http://www.fsbpt.org
This organization works to ensure that all physical thera-
    pists in the United States provide the same high level
    of service. It is responsible for the physical therapy
    national exam.

National Center for Complementary and Alternative
    Medicine
National Institutes of Health

9000 Rockville Pike
Bethesda, MD 20892
(888) 644-6226
Web site: http://www.nccam.nih.gov
The National Center for Complementary and Alternative
  Medicine conducts and supports research, trains comple-
  mentary and alternative medicine researchers, and
  provides information about such medicine.

New York Physical Therapy Association
5 Palisades Drive, Suite 330
Albany, NY 12205
(518) 459-4499
Web site: http://www.nypta.org
The NYPTA is a professional association working to improve
  health care for people of all ages and advancing physical
  therapy in the state of New York.

Ontario Physiotherapy Association
55 Eglinton Avenue East, Suite 210
Toronto, ON M4P 1G8
Canada
(800) 672-9668
Web site: http://www.opa.on.ca
The OPA is a health care organization for physiotherapists
  practicing in the province of Ontario. It provides
  career support services and opportunities for further
  education.

Sports Physical Therapy
201 S. Capitol Avenue, Suite 480
Indianapolis, IN 46225
(800) 285-7787
Web site: http://www.spts.org

The SPTS is a member of the American Physical Therapy Association. It provides a meeting place for those interested in sports physical therapy. Its mission is to provide the public and sports physical therapists with excellence in practice, research, education, and professional development.

U.S. Department of Labor
200 Constitution Avenue NW
Washington, DC 20210
(866) 4-USA-DOL (487-2365)
Web site: http://www.dol.gov
The Department of Labor works on behalf of job seekers, wage earners, and retirees of the United States by improving their working conditions and advancing their opportunities for profitable employment.

WEB SITES

Due to the changing nature of Internet links, Rosen Publishing has developed an online list of Web sites related to the subject of this book. This site is updated regularly. Please use this link to access the list:

http://www.rosenlinks.com/ecar/phys

for further reading

Burnet, James, and Andrew Long. *Getting into Physiotherapy Courses*. Richmond, Surrey, England: Trotman and Company, 2004.

Calabresi, Linda. *Human Body*. New York, NY: Simon & Schuster, 2008.

Curtis, Kathleen A. *The PTA Handbook: Keys to Success in School and Career for the Physical Therapist Assistant*. Thorofare, NJ: Slack, 2005.

Dawson, Ian. *Prehistoric and Egyptian Medicine*. New York, NY: Enchanted Lion Books, 2005.

Devantier, Alecia T., and Carol A. Turkington. *Extraordinary Jobs in Health and Science*. New York, NY: Ferguson, 2007.

Dreeben, Olga. *Introduction to Physical Therapy for Physical Therapy Assistants*. Sudbury, MA: Jones and Bartlett Publishers, 2006.

Esterson, Samuel H. *Starting & Managing Your Own Physical Therapy Practice: A Practical Guide for the Rookie Entrepreneur*. Sudbury, MA: Jones and Bartlett Publishers, 2005.

Exploring Health Care Careers. New York, NY: Ferguson, 2006.

Hawkins, Trisha. *Careers in Physical Therapy*. New York, NY: Rosen Publishing Group, 2001.

Horn, Geoffrey. *Sports Therapist*. Pleasantville, NY: Gareth Stevens, 2009.

Krumhansl, Bernice. *Opportunities in Physical Therapy Careers*. New York, NY: McGraw-Hill, 2005.

Langwith, Jacqueline. *Alternative Medicine*. Detroit, MI: Greenhaven Press, 2009.

Martin, Sieglinde. *Teaching Motor Skills to Children with Cerebral Palsy and Similar Movement Disorders: A Guide for Parents and Professionals*. Bethesda, MD: Woodbine House, 2006.

Pagliaro, Michael A. *Introduction to Physical Therapy*. St. Louis, MO: C. V. Mosby, 2001.

Porterfield, Deborah. *Top Careers in Two Years: Health Care, Medicine, and Science*. New York, NY: Ferguson, 2008.

Reeves, Diane Lindsey, Gail Karlitz, and Anna Prokos. *Career Ideas for Teens in Health Science*. New York, NY: Ferguson, 2005.

Vickery, Steve, and Marilyn Moffat. *The American Physical Therapy Association of Body Maintenance and Repair*. New York, NY: Owl Books, 1999.

Walker, Richard. *The Human Machine: An Owner's Guide to the Body*. New York, NY: Oxford University Press, 2008.

Woods, Michael, and Mary B. Woods. *The History of Medicine*. Minneapolis, MN: Twenty-First Century Books, 2006.

bibliography

All Allied Health Schools. "Physical Therapy Training Resources." Retrieved July 25, 2009 (http://www.allalliedhealthschools.com/faqs/physical_therapy).

Brissette, Sue. "Demographics: Shaping the Future of Physical Therapy." *PT in Motion*, June 2004. Retrieved July 16, 2009 (http://www.apta.org/AM/Template.cfm?Section=Archives3&TEMPLATE=/CM/HTMLDisplay.cfm&CONTENTID=8471).

Bureau of Labor Statistics. "Physical Therapists." *Occupational Outlook Handbook, 2008-09 Edition.* U.S. Department of Labor. Retrieved July 15, 2009 (http://www.bls.gov/oco/ocos080.htm).

Hawkins, Trisha. *Careers in Physical Therapy.* New York, NY: Rosen Publishing Group, 2001.

Inverarity, Laura. "Types of Physical Therapy." About.com, 2007. Retrieved July 3, 2009 (http://physicaltherapy.about.com/od/typesofphysicaltherapy/a/typesofpt.htm).

Jezek, Geno. "History of Magnets." HowMagnetsWork.com, 2006. Retrieved August 23, 2009 (http://www.howmagnetswork.com/history.html).

Memorial Hospital. "Physical Therapy." Retrieved August 1, 2009 (http://www.memorialhospital.org/PhysicialTherapySvcs.htm#balance).

Move Forward. "Why a Physical Therapist?" American Physical Therapy Association. Retrieved August 19, 2009 (http://www.moveforwardpt.com/why_physical_therapy).

Nemko, Marty. "Best Careers 2009: Physical Therapist." *U.S. News and World Report*, December 11, 2008.

Retrieved August 2, 2009 (http://www.usnews.com/
articles/business/best-careers/2008/12/11/best-careers-
2009-physical-therapist.html).

Office of the Professions. "Physical Therapy: License
Requirements." New York State Education Department.
Retrieved August 21, 2009 (http://www.op.nysed.gov/
ptlic.htm).

Science Daily. "Physical Therapy in ICU Can Reduce
Hospital Stays." October 24, 2007. Retrieved August 15,
2009 (http://www.sciencedaily.com/releases/2007/10/
071023164049.htm).

South Carolina Department of Labor, Licensing and
Regulation. "South Carolina Board of Physical Therapy."
Retrieved August 19, 2009 (http://www.llr.state.sc.us/Pol/
PhysicalTherapy/index.asp?file=ce.htm).

Walker, Emily. "Rising Obesity Rates Increases Nation's
Healthcare Tab." ABC News, July 27, 2009. Retrieved
August 1, 2009 (http://abcnews.go.com/Health/
WellnessNews/story?id=8185848&page=1).

index

About the Author

Though primarily an editor, Therese Harasymiw is the author of more than one hundred nonfiction children's books. She comes from a family of health care professionals, including doctors, nurses, and occupational therapists, all of whom were assets in the writing of this book. Harasymiw resides in Buffalo, New York, with her husband, Mark.

Photo Credits

Cover (left) © www.istockphoto.com/Pamela Burley; cover (right), p. 1 © www.istockphoto.com/Mads Abildgaard; pp. 4, 24–25, 47 © www.istockphoto.com; pp. 6, 21 © www.istockphoto.com/Eliza Snow; p. 10 © age fotostock/Superstock; p. 12 © www.istockphoto.com/Joseph Jean Rolland Dubé; pp. 14–15 © www.istockphoto.com/Pamela Moore; p. 18 © Véronique Burger/Photo Researchers; p. 26 © Lexington Herald-Leader/Zuma Press; p. 29 © Shutterstock; p. 30 © Courtesy of American Physical Therapy Association; pp. 34–35 © Contra Costa Times/Jose Carlos Fajardo/Zuma Press; p. 37 © www.istockphoto.com/Catherine Yeulet; pp. 40–41 © Steve Coddington/St. Petersburg Times/Zuma Press; p. 43 © A. Ramey/Photo Edit; pp. 48–49 © Scott Keeler/St. Petersburg Times/Zuma Press; pp. 52–53 © The Sacramento Bee/Dick Schmidt/Zuma Press; pp. 55 © www.istockphoto.com/Nancy Louie; p. 61 © www.istockphoto.com/Linda & Colin McKie; pp. 62–63 © BSIP/Phototake; pp. 64–65 © www.istockphoto.com/Mark Fairey.

Designer: Matt Cauli; Editor: Nicholas Croce; Photo Researcher: Marty Levick